Okay ...
Now What?

A Handbook for
New Cancer Parents

Pamela Chila Smith

ISBN: 978-1-960146-36-6 Hard Cover
        978-1-960146-37-3 Soft Cover

Chila. Pam Smith.

Edited by: Melissa Long

Warren publishing

Published by Warren Publishing
Charlotte, NC
www.warrenpublishing.net
Printed in the United States

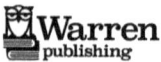

For My Nicky
I will forever keep the promises we made to each other.

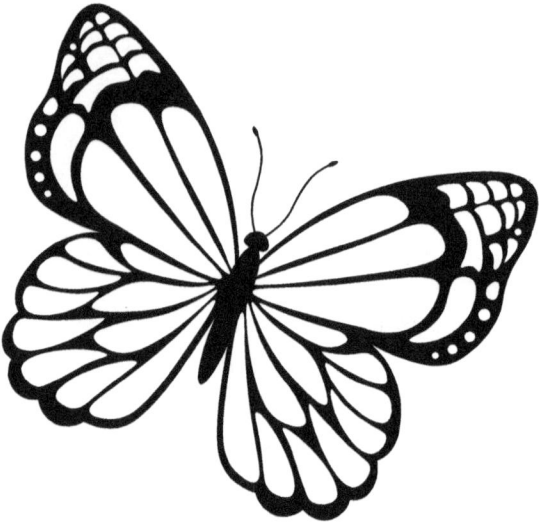

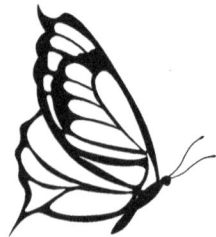

TABLE OF CONTENTS

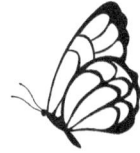

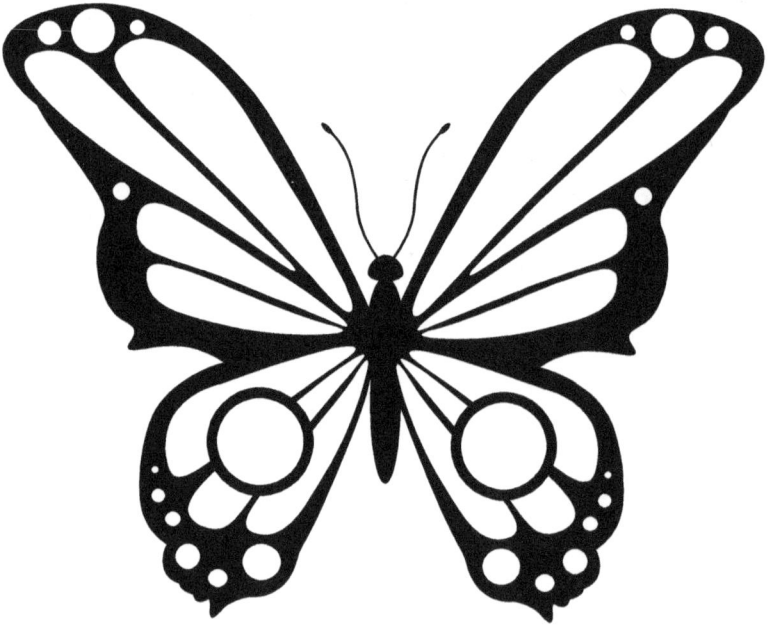

FOREWORD

Pam and I live in a world we wish on no other family — we both lost our sons to cancer. According to the CDC, as of this writing, about 15,000 children and adolescents younger than 20 years and over 21,000 young adults aged 20 to 30 years are diagnosed with cancer each year in the United States. The American Cancer Society says that after accidents, cancer is the second leading cause of death in children ages 1 to 14.

We are losing too many children.

In the years since my son Michael died, his father, brother and I have worked diligently to help other families, particularly on Long Island, NY, where a child has been diagnosed with cancer or other life-threatening chronic pediatric illnesses. The Michael Magro Foundation, a 501(c)3 non-profit organization, was established in January 2005 to honor Michael's life.

Pam wanted to and needed to write this book and we are grateful to be a part of her mission to help other families where their world has been turned upside down by their child's medical diagnosis.

We hope this handbook, with advice and personal stories, will help you better navigate the journey we wish you didn't have to take.

Terrie Magro
Michael Magro Foundation
www.MichaelMagroFoundation.com

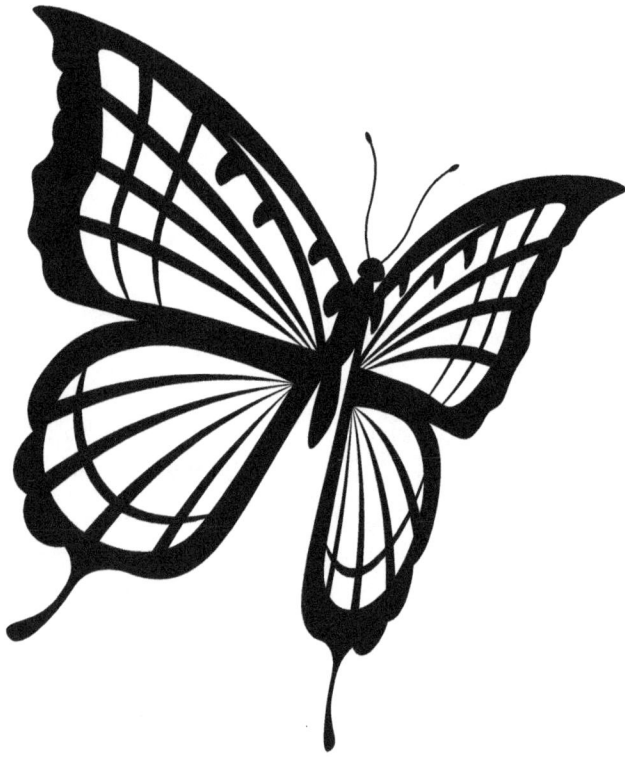

INTRODUCTION

Hi, I'm Pam, Nicholas's mom. In 2008, at fifteen years old, Nick was diagnosed with medulloblastoma, a type of brain cancer.

After weeks of progressive headaches, Nick and I finally had a quiet moment alone a few hours after his MRI had shown a brain tumor. We had been immediately been sent from our pediatrician's office to the ER of the local Children's Hospital to meet with the surgeon who would perform brain surgery the following morning. As I sat next to Nick's bed, I was handed a stack of paperwork and was told to read them. I rummaged through the pile of loose papers that were supposed to "help," but all I could think was, *Where do I start?*

I can still remember looking at Nick and saying, "Okay ... now what?"

He gave me his infamous shoulder shrug, and I put the papers to the side.

If you are reading this, then you have probably received some sort of medical diagnosis for your child. If you are thinking and asking the same questions I did, then I hope this book can help.

Throughout the book, I've broken things down into short paragraphs since things can get overwhelming extremely fast, and your head is going to spin enough from all that is being thrown at you. I wanted this to be more like a handbook, so I wrote it in a way where you can take your time, go straight to a chapter, or finish the whole book quickly.

Hopefully it will be easier to go to a specific subject. Short, simple, and to the point. The last thing you need is to be fumbling through a pile of paperwork. I used to toss those aside only to scramble through them later, hoping to find some type of information that might be helpful. In each chapter, I have also included some stories of my and Nick's own personal experiences.

By now the reality that your child is extremely sick may be starting to sink in. You may also be realizing you are now in charge of taking care of this devastating diagnosis. Your child needs you more now than ever before. They need you to keep it together and advocate. Fact is, caring for your child who has cancer has just become your full-time job. There are going to be good days, and there are going to be bad days. Unfortunately, you are going to have to be prepared for *all* days. This can be extremely hard.

It is a very scary word: *cancer.* It's even scarier when it's your own child. I'm sure we have all seen the commercials and thought to ourselves, *So sad, those poor kids,* then gone back to our normal lives. I will never forget the day when my son and I were sitting on the couch watching TV, not too long after chemo had started, and one of those very commercials came on. I looked at Nick, and he looked just like those kids, those beautiful, baldheaded kids who'd always brought me to tears. My worst nightmare, the reality of the situation, hit me at that moment.

It *can* happen to us. It *can* be your kid. It *was* my kid. It most definitely *is* scary.

So, As I said before, if you are reading this, then you have most likely received a diagnosis for your child. Please understand I am *not* an expert. I am just a mom who has lived this life. I am just like so many other cancer parents you may meet during this journey. Eventually, you will inherit the same title. Wear it proudly. It comes with a lot of blood, sweat, and tears.

As with everything new, it is going to take time to learn the coping mechanisms you are going to need. Go easy on yourself; it does not happen overnight! Life and experience will quickly teach you what you will need to know, so pay attention to what is going on around you. I will try to help as best as I can. Before you know it, you will be a pro. Although, I cannot tell you how to handle your particular situation. Everyone is different, but my goal is to give you some insight and guidance to help get you started on this pediatric cancer journey. Short and to the point.

Okay, ready? Here we go ....

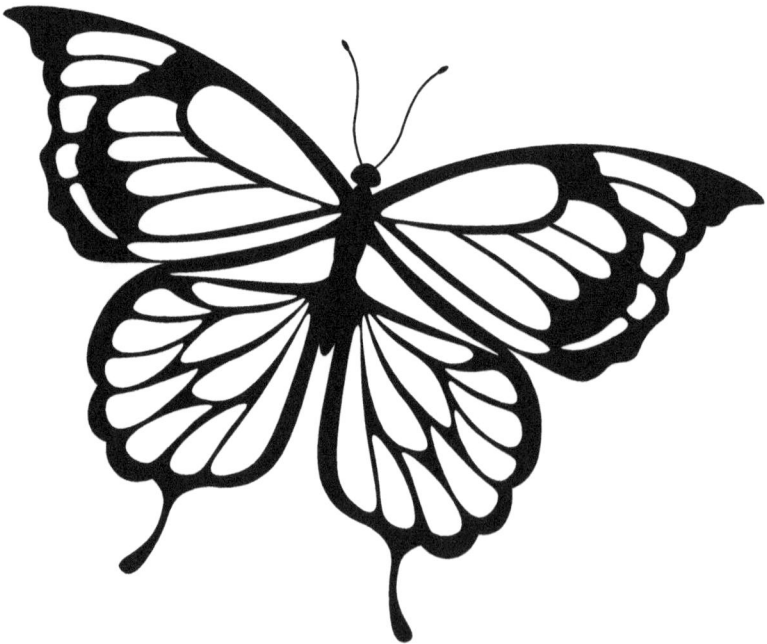

1.

GET A NOTEBOOK

The first thing I will advise you to do is to get yourself a notebook and pen. Always try to keep them with you or near you. Write everything down in that book. The date, what was discussed, questions you want to ask, procedures, names of medications, what dosage was given at what time. Log it all. It gives you something to look back on for reference.

Also, get a smaller book, one you can fit in your pocket and pocketbook. You are going to write all the medication information and any other significant information in it. Make sure to carry that one with you *always*. It is for emergency situations. It is extremely important to keep all information up to date. There will be, in most cases, a time where you will have to take your child to the emergency room and, possibly, to another hospital. This little book will be the one you will hand to the doctor when asked for information. It is easier than trying to remember it all, especially in an emergency. The book will have all the important information they will need. You will not have to worry about remembering it all, and you can focus on what is happening at that moment. Be prepared, whether you need it or not.

Start Writing

There are blank pages in the back of this book to get you started! Write down all the following information:

- The medication(s) your child is currently taking.
- The dosage next to each medication.
- The time each medication is given.
- All allergies your child has and if there is an allergy to any medications.
- Reactions to any type of specific medications.
- If your child has had chemotherapy and/or radiation.
- Your child's blood type.

*NOTE: Keep this information updated at all times!

2.

HOSPITAL BAG

This bag needs to be big enough to carry all your essentials. I, personally, used a large pocketbook big enough to hold everything. My laptop, notebooks, pens, snacks, folders for loose papers, change of clothes, cell phone chargers, toothbrushes, toothpaste, and more. It should *always* be packed. Use what works best for you. I can guarantee that at some point, you will need something from this bag. Be prepared to bring it with you or keep it nearby to be able to grab it and go. Remember, always be prepared.

Personal Story

My son was inpatient for most of 2009, and toward the end of our nine-month hospital stay, we had a resident who was new to our floor during his rotation. He was constantly making little comments about my books and how I never stopped writing in them to update the information. I always joked back about it.

A few months after I had gotten Nick home, I had to rush him to the emergency room due to seizures. Well, guess who came running into our room. That's right. It was that same resident! First thing he said was, "Where's your book?"

I pulled it out of my hospital bag—updated, packed, and ready to go at a moment's notice—and handed it to him.

He hugged me and apologized for teasing me. A few nurses came in that night and told me how having the information in front of them had saved time, and they were able to focus on Nick more quickly.

3.

ASK QUESTIONS

Now, you are going to feel every emotion possible. Don't worry. That's normal. The important thing is how you *use* those emotions. There is no time to sit in the why-my-child place. You have things to do. Start by getting ready to learn everything you can. Information is important. While I fully believe in researching things on your own, you will need to be careful when looking it up online. Yes, you will get a lot of information, but it does have the capability to give *too* much information. Some of it may not even pertain to your child's diagnosis, and the last thing you need is misinformation.

Ask the doctors, the nurses, the social worker, Child Life, or anyone on the floor you feel you can trust. Ask them everything. Even if you think it sounds foolish, ask anyway. From what chemotherapy will be given to what type of nausea medication works the best. What should you look out for with these medications, and are there side effects? What should you do if there is an allergic reaction? Ask questions until you feel you understand everything you want to know. And don't forget to write it all down.

Personal Story

It was the beginning of our battle, and we were in the hospital for about three days. Nick was sleeping comfortably, so I pulled out my laptop. Big mistake. I was looking up all the wrong information. I sat scrambling through all those loose papers and pamphlets for anything positive.

As I sat there, covered in all that mess and quietly sobbing, a PCA (Patient Care Aide) walked in. With all the kindness she could muster and a slight smile, she handed

me some tissues and gathered up all those papers I'd thrown around. Then she did me the biggest favor and took my laptop, saying it was dangerous right now to be looking for answers online, and proceeded to put it on the windowsill. She smiled and said it would be best to get the information from everyone who worked on the floor before going back online.

That night, I started writing my questions and answers in my little notebooks. That was the night I met Renee, who is someone I will forever consider family. She was there for me through it all, and I know she's still there if I need her now. I cherish her friendship.

4.

BUILD YOUR CANCER EMPIRE

Get advice. I talked to the other parents and the nurses—the ones who were hands-on, and the ones who have seen the most. They will be who you turn to. I honestly do not know what I would have done without them all. They were the greatest gifts we could've had through the whole illness.

Find your people. Start building your cancer empire. Ask for help! Your loved ones are there and willing. They are waiting for you to give them the word. They will become your shoulders to lean on. They will get you through the hard times.

You will be surprised though. There will be people who you thought would be there but are nowhere to be found. Then there are the unexpected ones who will step in and stay through it all. Try not get angry at those who remain silent or absent. You never know who has a legitimate excuse, like not being able (or knowing how) to handle your situation.

Pick someone to delegate. That person will reach out to those who want to help and give them things to do. Let that person take things off your shoulders. They can do things like plan dinners to have brought to your family, watch your other children if you have any, set up a CaringBridge account, or post on your social media. There are going to be extremely long days at the hospital and unexpected hospital stays. You are going to need help at a moment's notice. These are the people who will be there.

Personal Story

In February 2009, Nick took a turn for the worst. His treatments had been going relatively well up to this point. But the seizures had hit him hard, and this was when our real battle began. As a single mom at the time, knowing I could not be in the PICU (Pediatric ICU) with Nick and also care for my daughters who were just thirteen and eleven, Dawn, who was like a sister to me, drove fourteen hours to be with me and take care of my girls.

When Dawn had to go back home, my Aunt Sally did not miss a beat and stepped in to help. When we found out how severe Nick's condition was and realized he was not going home any time soon, my mom Linda stayed at my house for many months. Knowing she was there, and my girls were safe, I felt like I could breathe and focus on Nick. Unfortunately, my dad Jim had passed away two years earlier from cancer, so having my mom with us helped me emotionally as well, and I did not feel so alone. She is an amazing woman and I know I get my strength from her. I am so grateful and blessed to have her as my mom.

Having so much support from my family and friends meant everything to me. My empire included my friends Donna and Chris, Laura and Bob, Theresa and Jeff, Sandra and Kevin, Kathleen, Dawn and Chas, Trish and Jay, and so many more. My friend Bobby, Nick's soccer coach, had put together a fundraiser with Nick's soccer team. It was so incredible, we landed on our local news that night. Nick said he felt like a celebrity.

Winter in Long Island can be brutal. One morning, we woke up to quite a few inches of snow. I figured I'd get to shoveling after I fed everyone and gave Nick his medication. A little while later, my daughter called me to the front door to show me my neighbors had already started on the street and our driveway. They wanted to make sure we could get out or an ambulance could get through if we had an emergency. Truly the best neighbors.

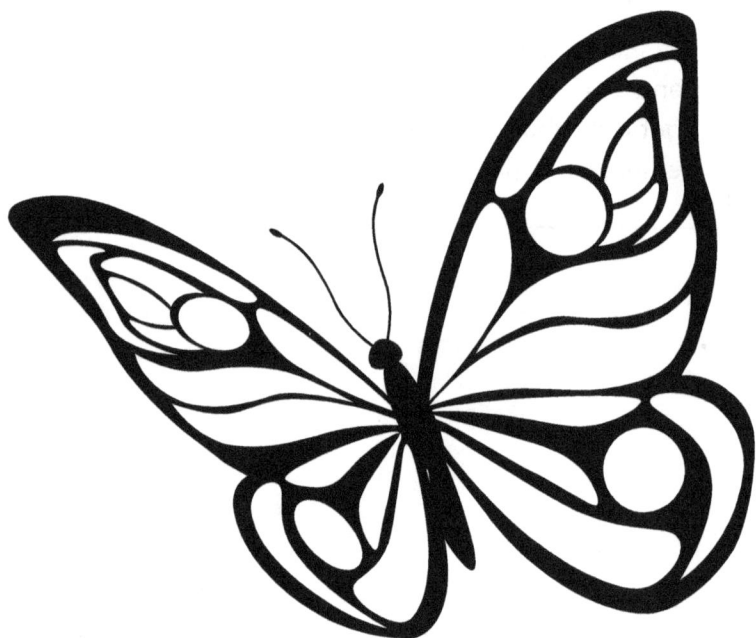

5.

YOUR CHILD IS A PERSON FIRST,
A DIAGNOSIS SECOND

Communication is the key to everything. First, listen to what your child is saying. Ask them how they are feeling, both physically and emotionally. Do this often. You need to make sure they are being heard by everyone involved, and their needs are being met. They are the important ones right now, and their voices should be heard above everyone else's.

It is so important to ask questions. *Lots* of questions. Write it all down in that notebook. Trust me, it will come in handy. If you do not understand what the doctors are saying, you have every right to ask for more information. This is *your* child, and you have every right to know what is going into their body.

Just to be clear, I am in no way saying you should refuse treatment. The doctors have the medicinal knowledge and should be trusted. They are doing what is in the best interest of your child, just like you are. What I am saying is everyone should be on the same page and working together. No one knows your child the way you do. The doctors will share with you what they feel is best, but it is also important for you discuss (not argue) with them any concerns you may have and what you feel is best for your child as well. Communication really goes a long way. If you have a difficult time with anyone, then you need to discuss it with someone you trust. Tell them you want all involved in a meeting to discuss the situation and resolve it. Calmly.

Personal Story

I did not get along very well with one of Nick's doctors. I did not like how he spoke to us; he came across very condescending, and we had a hard time communicating. Most of the time, I felt extremely frustrated and unheard with this particular doctor. He wanted to put Nick on a medication I was unsure about. I don't know how to explain it; my mom instincts just kept telling me "no." After a discussion, we agreed upon a small trial dose to see how he would handle it.

During that trial, one of our favorite doctors, Alyssa, whom we trusted completely, had popped in to say "hi" just in time for Nick to point out the window to show us the "blue dog running in the sky."

I asked, "A *what*?"

He said, "Look, Mom! There's a blue dog in the clouds."

He never took that medication again. I had another meeting with the care team and informed them I did not want the doctor I had been uncomfortable with treating Nick anymore. We had quite a few meetings, but we always walked out with things resolved. Nick was never treated by that doctor again. Alyssa, though, was amazing, and we adore her. She is kind and considerate, as well as smart. We communicated comfortably, and I knew she heard me. I could trust her and was able to talk to her about the good, the bad, and the ugly. She truly is the best.

6.

INNER VOICE

If you do not feel right about something, tell them! Listen to that inner voice we as moms, as parents, have. Doctors are just as human as you and I are; mistakes can and will happen. Your job is to try to stay on top of things and work together to catch them before something else does.

I am not ashamed to say I held my ground with a few doctors when my instincts were strong. There were times I somehow knew when something was wrong; you will not always be right, but those were the times I usually was. I knew my child. I made sure they saw him as a person. *My* child, *my* son, *my* life was lying in that bed. My job was to make sure he was not seen as a number on a file or a page in a medical book. This is where communication comes in handy. Call for meetings if necessary. Trust your instincts!

Personal Story

A few nights after my son had a shunt placed in his head to drain the excess brain fluid that developed, I could see by the way he was acting that something was wrong. There was a new fellow—a board-certified physician who had finished residency and was pursuing more specialized training in a specific area—this particular night, who repeatedly told me Nick was fine every time I called her in to check on him.

That was the night I found my voice.

After I loudly insisted Nick needed the shunt checked, the arrogant physician finally (reluctantly) placed a call to the brain surgeon, saying there was an "annoying mom insisting on a CT scan." Thankfully, the surgeon who was on that night told her to send him downstairs to have a scan done. It turned out his shunt had clogged, and his brain had too much fluid. The surgeon pulled an exorbitant amount of fluid out with a syringe through the shunt, and you could see the instant relief on my son's face. We brought him to the ICU, and he had surgery the next morning to replace the shunt. The surgeon told me that if I had not been so insistent, Nick would have died by morning.

The fellow obviously felt horrible and brought me a cup of coffee and sat with me at Nick's bedside that night. She promised to always listen to the parents and said this would never happen again. I hope she has kept her word.

Use your voice. Be heard.

7.

TAKE A MOMENT AND JUST BREATHE

There will be times when emotions will run extremely high, so it really helps to catch yourself in those moments. If you lose your temper or fall apart, it can all go wrong fast. At times, it is all going to get overwhelming. When it does, step away for a minute, take a breath, clear your head, then go back in with a clear, calm mind. Learn that early on; it helps.

Fight for your child, but do it respectfully.

Remember it is *never* okay to bully or physically handle anyone!

Believe me, you are going to have days and situations when you are going to want to explode. You will get too loud because we are human and scared and stressed. Just try not to let it get out of control. Nothing good comes from it. You can be firm. You can hold your ground during certain situations but do not allow things to escalate. Try to stay as calm as possible. Again, we know it is not an easy thing to do when you are trying to save your child's life. I have my own stories about this, but that is a totally different book!

Scream into a pillow if needed. I called my grandmother a lot. My MomMom, Connie, always knew what to say to calm me. If I did not want to talk then music helped. Get in your car and put the music on and sing loudly. You don't even have to leave your parking spot.

Stay calm. Take a moment. Just breathe.

Personal Story

One night, Nick and I were once again in the ICU and stable enough to go back up to the hemonc (hematology/oncology pediatric) floor. The problem this night was there were no open beds. The floor was full. When you have an immunocompromised child, you cannot just put them anywhere because the germs can kill them.

I had to hold my ground. There was a doctor and a nurse who were so angry because I would not do what they wanted, so we argued. They even called security on me. They were basically bullying me. I really hate bullies!

Security took me to a woman who was a higher-up, and as I began to tell her what was happening, as well as how I was being treated, she asked security to leave when she realized I wasn't a problem, just a concerned parent. She and I sat in her office as I explained what was going on, and she listened closely to everything I had to say. After a long, calm discussion, she and I finally came to an agreement hours later. She understood my refusal to put Nick in a regular hospital room with a sick, non-cancer child, so they put him in a thoroughly sanitized, private room until a bed became available on the cancer floor.

8.

KEEP THE LAUGHTER

Please, whatever you do, never show your child anything other than your "everything is okay" face. I have heard stories of children feeling guilty for being sick. They feel like they are at fault or putting everyone out because they need help. Make sure your child knows this is *not* their fault. Whenever I saw a certain look on my son's face, I would squeeze his hand and say, "It's all good," and he would relax. If he saw me stressed, he would do and say the same to me. Your child is more aware than you realize. Ease their fear as much as you can. They are scared and should not have to worry about you or anything else. Show them you have things under control. It takes so much pressure off them.

I had a strict rule throughout my son's illness: no one was to cry when they saw him. You would get escorted out of his room and away from him if you did, and, yes, I walked a few people out. He was to know only the smiles and the laughter. He had enough to deal with. He did not need to see everyone blubbering like fools. Everyone was respectful and walked in with a smile. Our family always says we laughed our way through cancer.

The focus is to keep your child as positive as possible. Do not let cancer steal those precious, priceless moments. Do not let it steal the laughter. As hard as it is, keep smiling at them. Keep them calm. Their only job is to heal. Your job is everything else.

Personal Story

Nick and I laughed *a lot*! He felt like himself when it was a lighter, fun atmosphere. Almost like he was not sick. Nick had a nurse named Melissa, and he absolutely adored her, and the feeling was mutual. They had an instant connection, especially since her sense of humor matched his. Best buds; two peas in a pod. He found it funny to call the nurses station when things were quiet, just to see where she was. I had to keep him from yelling her name when she was nowhere to be found. They had some bond.

One day, Nick dared his sister Jen and Nurse Melissa to go all the way downstairs into the middle of the hospital lobby and dance. I can still see the look of shock and delight on his face when they ran for the elevator. Nick, my daughter Michelle, and I went to the hallway where we could see them dancing away in the lobby. The whole thing made him laugh hysterically. I still have the pictures.

On a side note, during the fun times and the not-so-fun times, Melissa was always professional and took incredible care of him, right to the end. I am eternally grateful to and for her, and she will always be a part of our family. Could not have made it through without her.

9.

DON'T LEAVE YOUR CHILD ALONE

I t is so very important that someone stays with your child at all times!
No child should be left alone during a cancer battle. Especially when
they are admitted into the hospital. Not only can it be extremely
scary for them, but also something could happen while they are alone
that puts their life at risk. If you need to step out briefly, to grab coffee
or food, that is not a big deal, but getting into your car and leaving for
a few hours is not advisable. As I have said before, this diagnosis is *your*
responsibility. Your child is already battling a disease that is trying to
take over their body. They are dealing with enough.

Something else I feel is so important, whether your child is in the
hospital or not, is that the doctors should be talking to you exclusively
about your child's care, not your child. Make that clear to your child and
the doctors. In some hospitals, doctors will go into the hospital room
and talk directly to your child if no one is there. *No* decision should be
made or agreed upon by a minor. Decisions should always be made by
or with an adult present. Make it clear to whomever walks into your
child's room that they are to talk to only you, not to your child, at all.
It is scary for a teenager, so it must be petrifying to a young child.

I cannot stress this enough: *stay* with your child and be their voice.

Personal Story

Our doctors on the hemonc floor were good when they came into the room to talk to the parents. They respected us when we asked them not to go directly to Nick. Every now and then, if there was a new doctor, or we were on a different floor, I would notice they would talk to Nick like I was not there.

One night, the nurse walked in and started to discuss medication with him. I had to ask her to talk to *both* of us. He was a minor with brain cancer, and he did not want them talking to him alone. He always said he felt safer not making the decisions. He was sixteen at the time. He was never left alone, especially after he voiced his concerns. After I told her how he felt, she talked to us both.

10.

MEDICATION AND PAIN

B e aware of when all medication should be given. *Always* stay ahead of the pain! If you get caught behind it, it will be difficult to catch up. In other words, make sure medications *do not* wear off! You do not want your child in any kind of pain. If you are in the hospital and noticing it is almost time for the next dose, you can let the nurse know even if they are usually on top of things. They will understand and are often happy to help. In our situation, I can honestly say, I could not have gotten through it all without the group of people we had at our hospital. They were amazing.

If your child is ever experiencing more pain than normal, make sure you inform someone *immediately*. Any changes need to be looked at as soon as possible. If there is anything that does not seem right, talk to the doctors as soon as possible. If you are home, call them. If you are in the hospital, have the doctor come to the room and physically check on your child. You can never be too safe when it comes to your child's life. Again, *no one* knows your child the way you do.

Push the issue if you are feeling like you are not being heard!

Advocate!

Make them *hear* you!

Personal Story

Nick often battled with seizures controlled through medication. We had to stay on top of his dosage constantly. His medication had to be given on time, or we could throw him into a seizure easily. If his dose was too low, that could also be a problem.

When we were in the Bone Marrow Transplant Unit, I explained this to the new doctor who seemed to just smile and "okay" me.

I said again that Nick *needed* to have his full dosage, or he would seize. She ordered for his medication to be chopped up and pushed through his NG (nasogastric) tube.

I brought up once again that he would not get the full dosage that way because it would stick to the inside of the tube, and there was a liquid form she should use instead. She said it would be fine.

Completely frustrated, I warned her *again* that he would seize. She just smiled at me.

He seized.

I called our neurosurgeon, who always helped when the shunt clogged, and explained what was going on. She ordered the liquid and called the bone marrow specialist. Guess who walked in and informed me that *she* spoke to neurology and was putting him on the liquid form? I was fuming, so I called a meeting. We had very big discussion at that meeting. I voiced how she was not listening to me, and I was the one who called neurology to explain the situation. In the end, she finally agreed to work together and said she would listen when I spoke of my son's needs. It was a much-needed and productive meeting. Thankfully, we had a good relationship from there on.

Mutual respect and communication is so very important.

11.

FINANCES

For most of us, this will hit hard. *Really* hard.

As I mentioned before, I strongly advise there be at least one parent, or guardian, with your child always. This usually leaves one parent to work or alternate their shifts. One income, for most people in this day and age, is extremely difficult but unavoidable during this battle. If you are lucky enough to be financially stable with one income, consider yourself blessed. That is a *huge* stress you will not have to endure quite as painfully as those less fortunate.

Unfortunately, especially for those of us who are single parents, it adds an enormous amount of stress on top of what we are already going through. Ask for help when needed. There will be organizations available and offering to help. Accept it. Do *not* let your pride get the better of you. Trust me, take all the help that is offered. There are foundations available for just this reason. They are formed from families who have been in the same situation.

People are generous and want to help. The nicest feeling is someone handing you a hot meal they made for your family, especially after a really long day at the hospital. Gift cards are fantastic also.

Personal Story

After Nick was diagnosed, and I left work to care for him full-time, things were extremely tight financially. I remember thinking, *How am I going to juggle the bills and feed us?*

After the mortgage was paid, there was very little money left for the entire month. I tell you what, I am grateful for the companies who accepted late payments with no penalty fees. Usually, companies are understanding and willing to help during times like these. The hospital's breakfast cart kept me from starving, but the foundations helped the most! The hospital will be able to provide you with information for all the local foundations.

I was always so thankful for incredibly generous family and friends. If anyone asks what you need, tell them, "Gift cards!" Gift cards saved me on many occasions. One of the greatest gifts I got from my friends Jeanne and John were gas gift cards so I could easily fill up my vehicle. When you have nothing in the bank and are riding on empty while trying to get to and from the hospital, it is a relief to have them.

12.

MARRIED PARENTS AND PARTNERS

For those parents who are married, the stress and worry that comes with the diagnosis can cause even the most solid relationships to turn bitter. I know this is a difficult time for you both, but *do not* turn on each other. When you're scared and angry, it is so easy to take it out on the person closest to you.

Who else can you do that to, right?

Wrong!

Try not to let it get too far. There have been many couples who were not able to recuperate from things said in the heat of the moment. Trust me, there will be a lot of those moments, but you can't let them separate or break you. Let this diagnosis bring you together, make you stronger. You are both fighting the same battle. Remain teammates. Partners. Lean on each other. Your child needs to see you are all in this together.

For those who are not legally married but are in a relationship, the same thing applies. Whether it is your child or your significant other's child, you are in this *together*. You will need to be just as supportive and understanding. Be a team.

Personal Story

My now-husband Ken and I are childhood friends. We reconnected when Nick was nearing the end of his battle.

Kenny and Nick clicked right from the start, which was a huge relief! Nick had always dreamed of being a pilot. He also wanted to join the Air Force. When Nick found out that Kenny had been in the Air Force when he was younger, Nick was ecstatic. They talked and joked constantly. Poor Nick lived in a house with all women and would call Kenny, saying he was "drowning in an estrogen ocean." This would cause us all to start laughing so loud, it filled the house, especially when Nick would yell, "Please visit and bring more testosterone to the house!" Those moments are my most favorite memories. Listening to the man I love joke and laugh with my children is something I will cherish forever. The way he loves me and my children, and now we have our son Benjamin ... to say I am blessed is an understatement.

He is my rock. He makes me laugh and is my shoulder to cry on. He listens when I need to talk and picks up the pieces when I am falling apart. He also reminds me to breathe when I feel like I can't. He is truly my partner.

13.

DIVORCED PARENTS

For those parents who are divorced, you may or may not be on very good terms, so be prepared because you are now going to be thrown together into an extremely stressful situation. Put your differences aside, *immediately*. As of now, those differences and any issues you may have no longer exist. This is not about either of you; it is about the child you have together. You have just become partners again. Figure out how to work together and find that common ground. The importance of that is extraordinary. It will not always be easy for either of you, but this is something you have got to make work. There is something much bigger to fight now, and the last thing your child needs is to see you two fighting with each other. This situation doesn't call for any type of unnecessary drama. Remember why you are here. Your child needs you to be a united front.

Personal Story

The morning after we found Nick's tumor, he was heading into surgery when my phone started ringing like crazy. My sister Doreen was on her way to the airport to pick up our mom, and they would be to the hospital soon. I was somehow still breathing, although it felt like I was trapped in a nightmare. I wanted someone to wake me up. My two high school best friends came running to support me. While my friend Sandy was driving in from Virginia, my friend Kathleen brought me supplies and helped me freshen up in the waiting-room restroom.

I vaguely remember everyone arriving, but eventually, our big, divorced family all came together in that waiting room. We stood at Nick's bedside eight-and-a-half hours later. He was waking up, and even though his eyes had not even opened yet, he was already making us all laugh.

As part of a divorced family, I am extremely proud of the way we as parents come together for our children. Our family works very well together through even the toughest of crises. We just somehow drop our defenses and team up.

Is it always easy? No.

Do we put our children above everything? Yes.

I remember this one day when we were all gathered in Nick's room. We must have been loud because my friend Lisa, whose daughter Carly was inpatient in the room next to us, stopped me at the nurses station later that evening and asked if all that noise was us. I apologized, feeling embarrassed, but she said it was nice to hear all the laughter coming out of his room. It makes me smile to think that even though he was so sick, Nick was surrounded by his family in a happy and an uplifting way.

Really quick, I want to say how grateful I am to Nick's grandparents. His Grandma Jean was with us every day and was an incredible support for me. I carry my time with her and his Grandpa Jerry in my heart always.

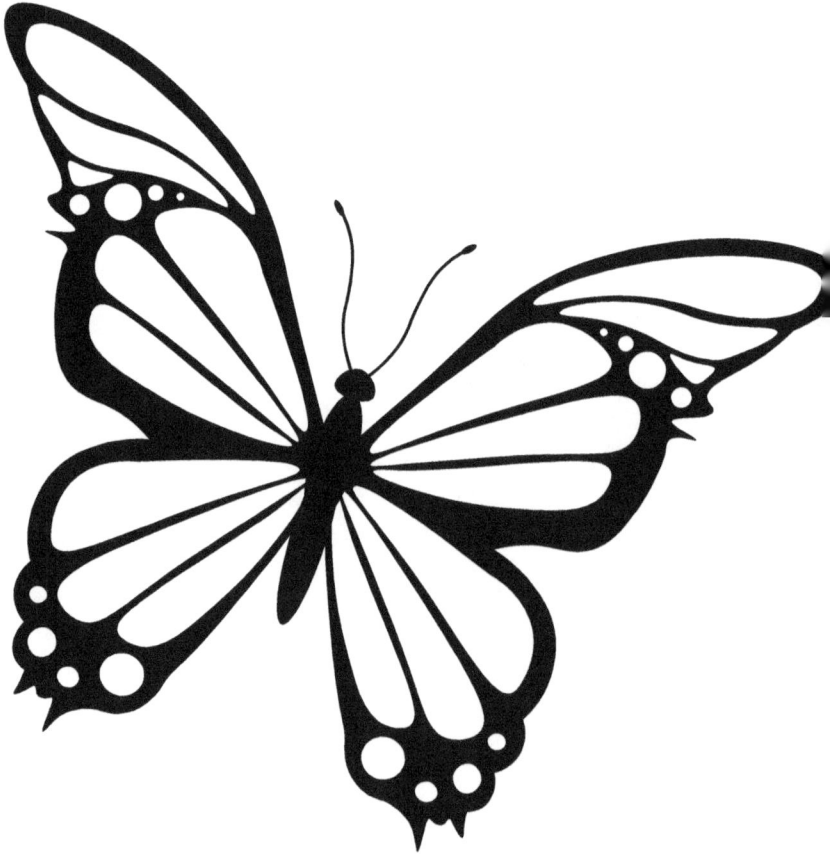

14.

SIBLINGS

This is so important for parents with more than one child! Please remember they are just as shocked and overwhelmed as you are. Their lives have just turned upside down too. Siblings are usually very close, and it can be hard when one of them is sick. It can make the healthier siblings extremely scared, or they may want to help take care of them. Most of the time, it is both. Talk to them but, more importantly, *listen* to them. Listen to their needs and their fears. Just know what they will need is stability, support, and a loving place to be able to go to on a moment's notice where they will find comfort.

This is where you will need to ask for help. You cannot be in two places at once, and unfortunately, cancer outranks everything right now. You will need as many supportive people as you can get. Your children will get moved around quite a bit due to doctor's appointments or hospital stays. You will need some assistance. Treatments can take hours or, at times, all day. Have people whom you trust to take care of them when you cannot be there.

Please, whatever you do, make sure they *do not* feel abandoned or forgotten. When it is possible, make sure to have some one-on-one time. A quick lunch alone or even a simple "I'm thinking about you" or

"I love you" text will suffice. Any type of contact that lets them know you are there for them too.

If they are old enough, keep them involved. Most will want to feel they are a part of what is going on. Siblings have a strong bond. Let them spend time together. It is good for all of you to maintain that family closeness.

Personal Story

My kids were at the hospital a lot, especially Nick's sister Michelle. They even missed school if they felt it was important to be with their brother for the day, and that was fine with me. I did not know what the outcome would be for Nick, but just in case, I wanted them to spend as much time together as possible.

They made so many memories during that time. The kids still remember the stories and the laughter. They took so many pictures and treasure every one of them now. There was one day when I did not bring my daughter Michelle because she had a test that day. Unfortunately for her, when I arrived at the hospital, her favorite singer at the time was performing in the lobby. I hated having to tell her she missed Justin Bieber because she was so bummed. Child Life did manage to get her a hat at least, so I took a picture of Nick wearing it and sent it to her. I never said "no" again when she asked to go with me.

When my son Matthew would go to the hospital to watch football, it was always such a big deal to Nick. He would wait for Matt, wearing all his New York Giants apparel, his jersey and hat, which was always backward. See, Matt's a New York Jets fan and would show up wearing *his* team. Game on!

My daughter Jen would do whatever she could to make Nick smile. If there was a hospital gown in her reach, she would wrap her head in it. The moment Nick would turn around and see her, he would let out a loud belly laugh. When we finally got him home, she would carry him anywhere he wanted to go.

Lots of pictures and videos were taken. Siblings really are the best medicine!

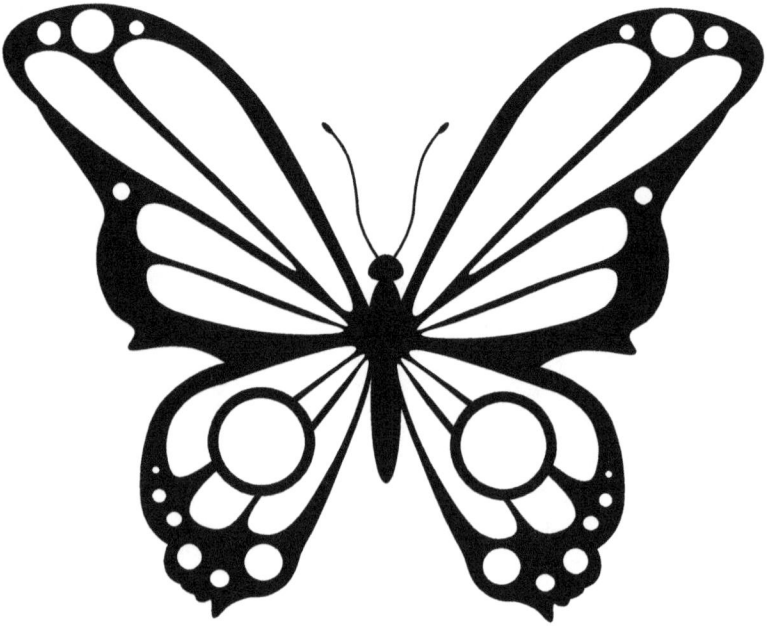

15.
MAKE MEMORIES

You think this cancer experience is something you are going to want to forget, but the crazy thing is you will want to remember more than you realize.

Take those pictures and videos of both the good and bad moments. Make those memories you will later look back on with a smile or a tear but also with a whole new perspective. It will go hand-in-hand with those books you are logging everything in. Write things you think you may want to remember, and if you are not sure … well, write them anyway! You will be surprised and happy you did.

Personal Story

I have always been a picture taker. At a young age, my Aunt RoseMarie said to me, "They aren't pictures, they're memories." I think I have always lived by that phrase. I have an astronomical amount of pictures of my children in every phase of their lives. When they introduce me to people, like friends and such, they always say, "This is my mom, the tourist. She will take your picture before you leave the room." Yes, I am guilty of that.

When I brought Nick home from the hospital, after he was inpatient for nine months, my goal was to make as many memories as possible. His buddies Steve, Scott, Zack, and Liz came over often. There was a lot of pizza and laughter, and there were a lot of pictures taken. Coach Bob put together a luncheon with the soccer team, and Nick was over the moon. More pictures, more memories.

You see, the doctors offered us the option of doing five weeks of additional radiation. I asked how much more time that would give us. They said maybe an extra two weeks. "So," I said, "we would be putting him through five weeks of pain for maybe two weeks more?" Or I could bring him home and enjoy the time we had left. I obviously told them "no."

Then I took him home, and we made some pretty great memories.

I still have the pictures to prove it.

16.

KEEP THE FAITH

I hope this was of some help for you. You will not walk away from this experience the same person you were when it began. Find your inner strength and use your voice. If given the opportunity, be a help to others. This is the most difficult path you will ever walk down, but you will find the strength to do it.

I wish I could tell you there are always happy endings. For some, there are. And for others, like my son Nicholas, there are not.

For a year and nine months, we could not have fought any harder than we did during that time. In 2010, my Nicky passed away peacefully in my arms, surrounded by his family and his favorite nurse Melissa in our home. I miss him more with every breath I take.

I wrote this handbook to honor my amazing son and his strength during his battle. I am hoping that by sharing what I learned through our fight, I can somehow help you. My prayers are with you, and may your family have a happier, healthier ending. Stay strong, keep the fight and the faith. Don't forget to just breathe.

From Nick and I, "It's all good."

Blessings to you and your family from me and my family,
Pam

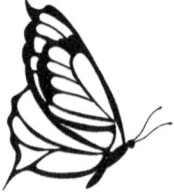

ACKNOWLEDGMENTS

To my husband, Ken and my children, Matthew, Nicholas, Jennifer, Michelle, and Benjamin, you are my moon and my stars.

To my mom, Linda, and my sister, Doreen, as well as all our Family and Friends.

To Harley Belle and Haizley , Nana Loves you.

To our amazing nurses and doctors who took incredible care of Nick.

To my Cancer Mom's and our Angels and Survivors, who walked those halls with me.

To Terrie from the Michael Magro Foundation and Lori, for your support and for believing in me. Our boys would be proud of us.

To Mindy, Amy, and Melissa from Warren Publishing, for helping me put a promise into print.

With all my heart... Thank You.

NOTES

_____

_____

_____

_____

_____

_____

_____

_____

_____

_____

_____

_____

_____

_____

_____

_____

_____

_____

_____

NOTES

NOTES

NOTES

NOTES

NOTES

NOTES

NOTES

NOTES

NOTES

NOTES

_____

_____

_____

_____

_____

_____

_____

_____

_____

_____

_____

_____

_____

_____

_____

_____

NOTES

NOTES

NOTES

NOTES

NOTES

NOTES

_____

_____

_____

_____

_____

_____

_____

_____

_____

_____

_____

_____

_____

_____

_____

_____

_____

NOTES

NOTES

_____

_____

_____

_____

_____

_____

_____

_____

_____

_____

_____

_____

_____

_____

_____

_____

NOTES

NOTES

NOTES

NOTES

NOTES

NOTES

NOTES

NOTES

NOTES

NOTES

NOTES

NOTES

NOTES

_____
_____
_____
_____
_____
_____
_____
_____
_____
_____
_____
_____
_____
_____
_____
_____
_____
_____
_____

NOTES

NOTES

NOTES

NOTES

NOTES

NOTES

NOTES

NOTES

NOTES

NOTES

NOTES

NOTES

NOTES

NOTES

NOTES

NOTES

NOTES

NOTES

NOTES

NOTES

NOTES

NOTES

NOTES

NOTES

NOTES

NOTES

NOTES

NOTES

www.ingramcontent.com/pod-product-compliance
Lightning Source LLC
Chambersburg PA
CBHW022340280326
41934CB00006B/716